8/00

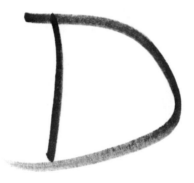

The Let's Talk Library™

Let's Talk About Having the Flu

Elizabeth Weitzman

The Rosen Publishing Group's
PowerKids Press™
New York

Published in 1997 by The Rosen Publishing Group, Inc.
29 East 21st Street, New York, NY 10010

Copyright © 1997 by The Rosen Publishing Group, Inc.

First Edition

Book Design: Erin McKenna

Photo Illustrations: Front cover by Carrie Ann Grippo; pp. 4, 8, 11, 12, 15, 16, 19, 20 by Carrie Ann Grippo; p. 7 © 1992 J. L. Carson/Custom Medical Stock.

Weitzman, Elizabeth.
    Let's talk about having the flu / Elizabeth Weitzman.
        p.   cm. — (The Let's talk library)
    Includes index.
    Summary: Explains what causes the flu, how you feel when you have it, and what can be done to treat this disease.
    ISBN 0-8239-5030-1 (lib.bdg.)
    1. Influenza—Juvenile literature. [1. Influenza. 2. Diseases.]   I. Title. II. Series.
    RC150.W33 1996
    616.2'03—dc20   96-43325
                                                                                CIP
                                                                                AC

Manufactured in the United States of America

Contents

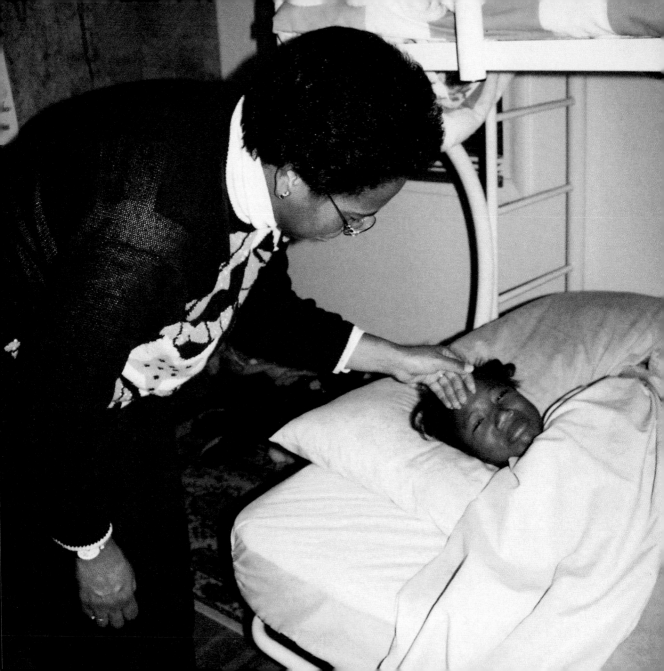

Daria

Daria came downstairs to breakfast with a red nose and watery eyes. "Are you feeling okay?" her mother asked. Daria shook her head and sneezed. "My head hurts. And I'm cold," she answered. Her mother felt her forehead. "You may be cold, but you feel very warm to me." She gave Daria some orange juice. "Go back upstairs and get in bed," she said. "It looks like you've caught the flu."

◄ Having the flu is not fun, but you will not feel bad for very long.

What Is the Flu?

Most of the time, your body protects itself from unhealthy **germs** (JERMZ). Germs are living things that are so tiny that thousands can fit on the tip of a pencil. A **virus** (VY-rus) is a type of germ that can cause many illnesses. The flu, also called **influenza** (in-floo-EN-za), is one of these illnesses. Having the flu feels like having a very bad cold. People often get the flu during the winter.

A virus is made of many tiny living things called germs. ▶

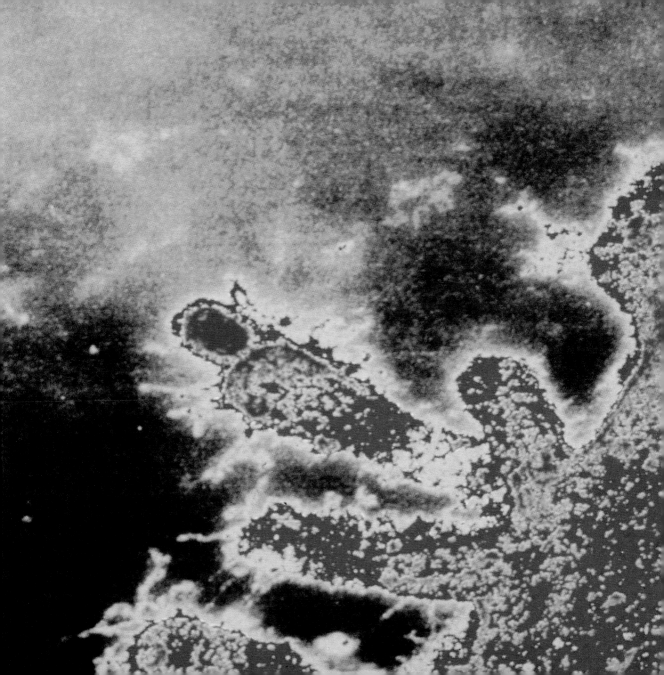

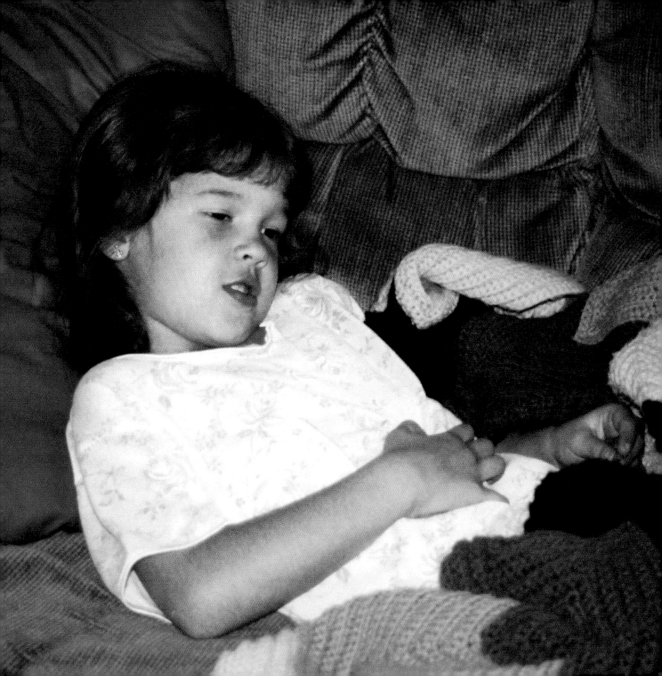

How Do You Feel?

When you have the flu, you feel pretty bad. Some people get headaches or stomachaches. Most people get a **fever** (FEE-ver). And just about everyone has a runny or stuffy nose. The flu makes you sneeze and cough a lot. It's no fun being sick. However, it might help to remember that the flu only lasts about one week.

◄ A person with the flu may have a stomachache and feel very tired.

Why Do You Feel So Bad?

Once the flu virus is inside you, your body tries to fight it. Believe it or not, *that's* what makes you feel bad. Your **temperature** (TEMP-rah-chur) rises to kill the germs. That gives you a fever. Extra blood goes to the area around your eyes and nose, so you feel stuffy. Your nose makes more **mucous** (MYOO-kus) than usual, which gives you a runny nose.

A fever when you are sick means that your body is fighting germs. ▶

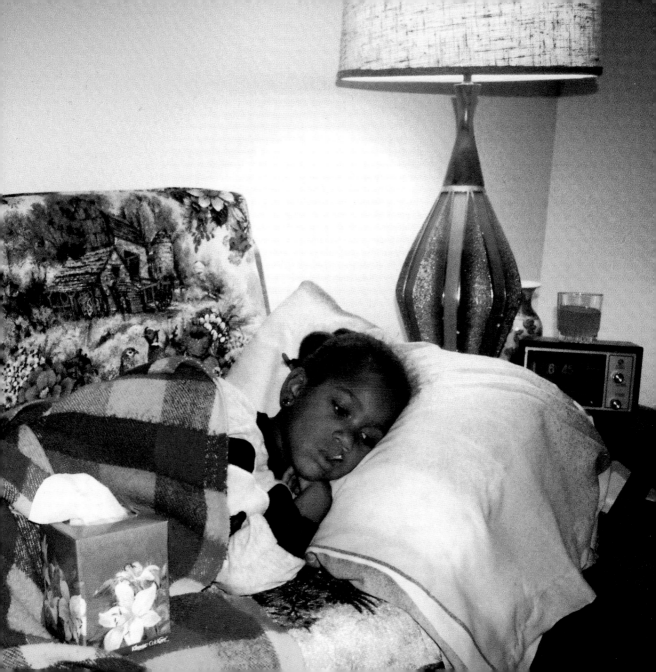

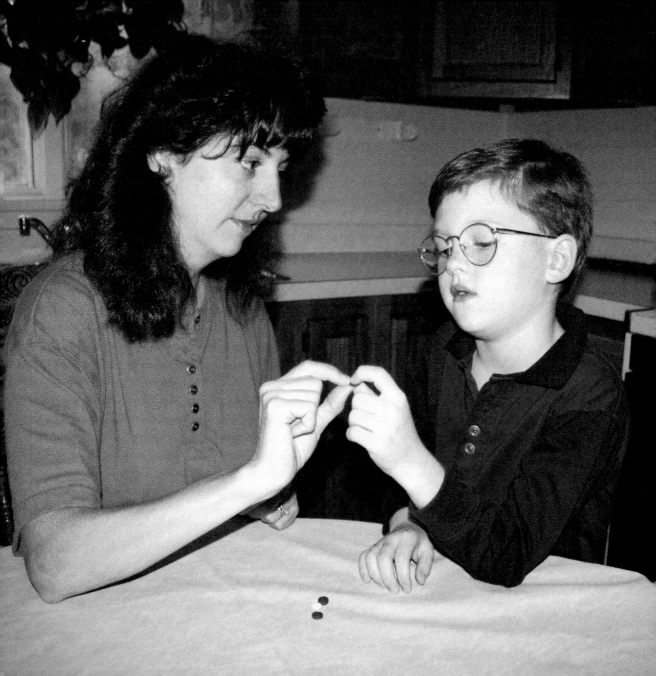

How Can You Feel Better?

There's no medicine that cures the flu. But there are things that will make you feel better. First, stay in bed. Sleep and rest are good for your body when you're sick. Second, drink lots of water and juice. Your body needs the extra **fluids** (FLOO-ids). Your mom or dad may give you some medicine to help your head or nose to feel better for a while.

◀ A grown-up can give you some medicine to help you feel better.

Stay in Bed!

It is important to rest when you have the flu. Most of the time, you won't feel like doing much anyway. But there's no need to be bored just because you have to stay in bed. There are toys you can play with while you're in bed. Ask your mom if she can take out some books from the library for you. One of your friends may be able to bring over your schoolwork, too.

There are lots of things to do in bed while you are getting over the flu. ▶

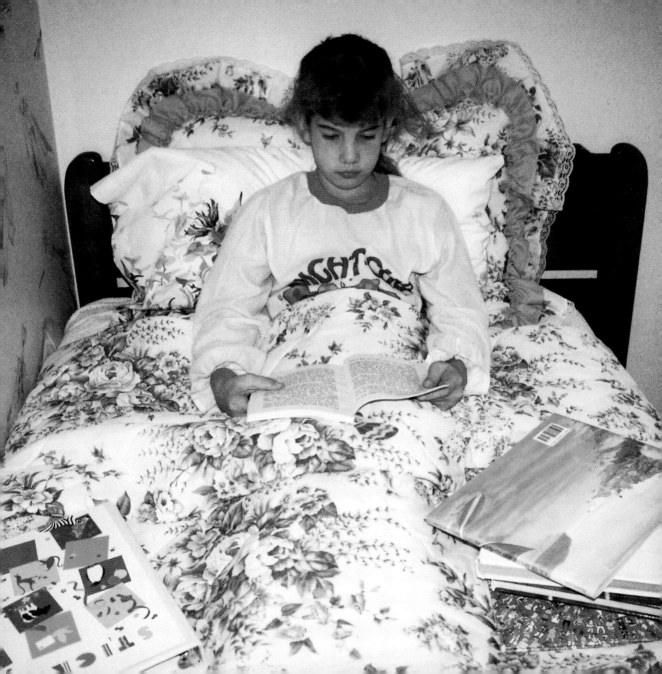

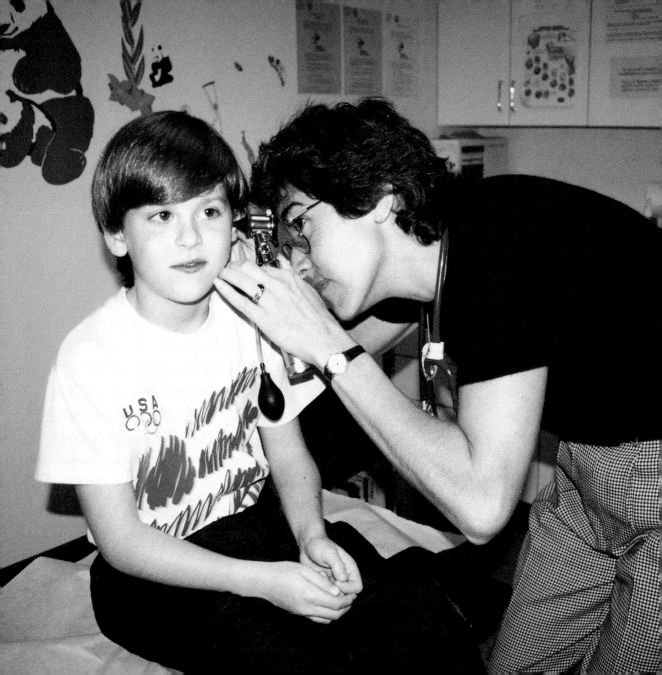

Going to the Doctor

Your parents may decide you should see a doctor. The doctor will make sure that you really have the flu. She may take your temperature, just like your parents do. She will probably ask you to open your mouth really wide so she can look at your throat. She will also check your ears and your chest. None of these things hurt, so there's no need to be scared or nervous.

◀ The doctor will check very carefully to see if you have the flu.

How Can You Avoid the Flu?

Flu germs enter your body through your nose, eyes, and mouth. Usually, you pick them up from the air or things you touch. To help keep yourself from getting the flu, always wash your hands before you eat. And try not to rub your eyes and nose. Also, remember to cover your mouth when you sneeze or cough, especially if you have the flu. And it's not a good idea to share food or drinks when you're sick.

Protect yourself from germs by washing ▶
your hands before meals.

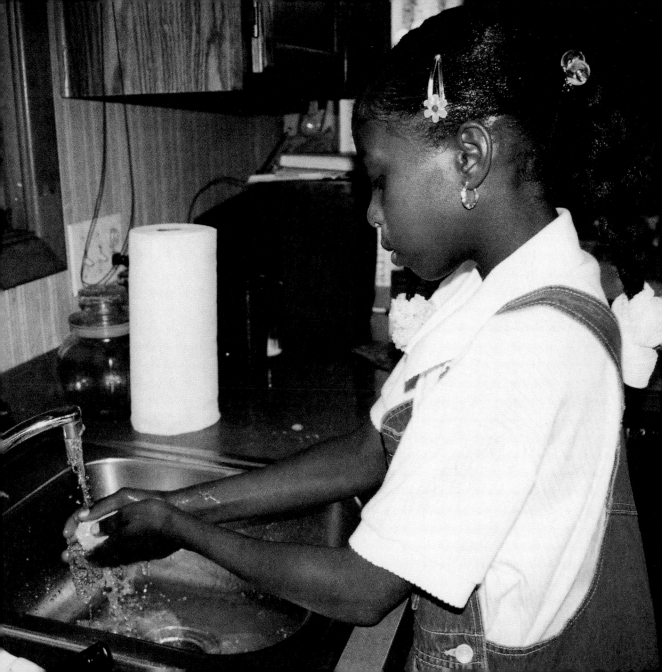

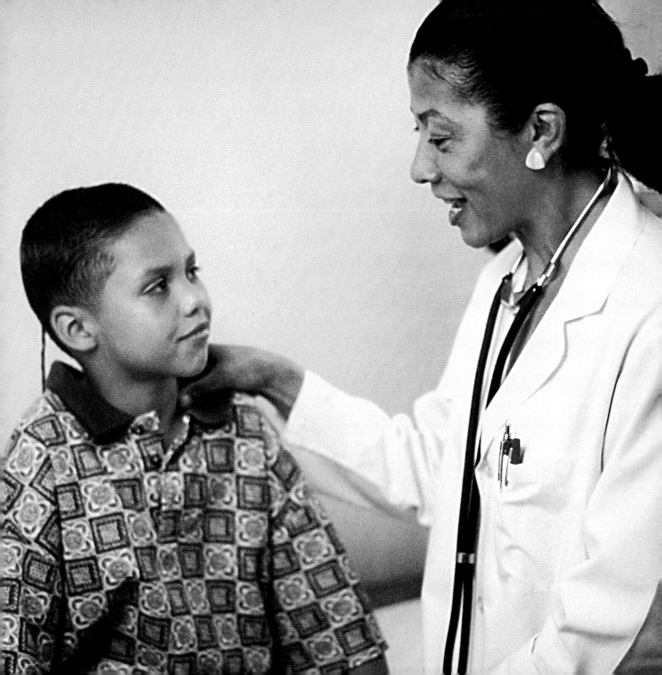

Flu Vaccine

There is another way to protect yourself from the flu. Your doctor may want you to get a flu **vaccine** (vax-EEN) at the beginning of the winter. A vaccine is usually given as a shot. The shot feels like a strong pinch, but it's over quickly. A vaccine puts a tiny amount of the flu virus in your body. The amount is so small it doesn't make you sick. But your body learns how to fight these germs. Your body will know how to fight more germs of the same kind.

◄ The doctor will tell you that the shot may hurt for a little while, but the flu vaccine can help your body fight the flu virus.

You'll Feel Better Soon

Everyone gets the flu at some time. It might help to remember that the aches and pains are just your body's way of fighting the bad germs inside you. Get lots of rest and drink plenty of fluids. And no matter how bad you feel, don't forget that the flu only lasts about five to ten days. After that, you should be back on your feet and feeling great again!

Glossary

fever (FEE-ver) A rise in your body heat.
fluid (FLOO-id) Liquid.
germ (JERM) Tiny living thing that can cause
  sickness.
influenza (in-floo-EN-za) The flu.
mucous (MYOO-kus) A thick liquid that forms in
  your nose and throat during a cold.
temperature (TEMP-rah-chur) How hot or cold
  something is.
vaccine (vax-EEN) A protection against a sickness,
  usually given as a shot.
virus (VY-rus) A type of germ.

Index